Recipes:

I0407746

GREENS, DETOX & SMOOTHIES

Weight Loss and Healthy Living

Joanne Howard

Table of Contents

Introduction

It is very sad that even though we know how important it is to take fruits and vegetables, we still don't take as much of these foods as we should. This has led to nutrient deficiencies. One of the ways that these deficiencies manifest themselves is our need to overeat because the body is looking for how to get the nutrients that it desperately needs. As we give in to our urges, we are likely to want to take highly processed foods, which in most instances are high in artificial substances. This leads to high toxin levels, unnecessary weight gain and a plethora of other problems. If you want to live a long and healthy life, you have to eat more fruits and vegetables. Since most of us do not like the taste of vegetables especially when cooked, why not mix the vegetables and fruits in a juice. This way, you take your daily requirements of both fruits and vegetables and you don't have to gag to that awful taste of broccoli for instance.

This book will provide you with amazing juicing recipes today that you can try out for a healthier you. The recipes are really simple; you can actually have most of the juices ready in less than 15 minutes. How cool is that? Well, if you really want to lose weight, feel energetic and just amazing, you can bet that this book is your express ticket to achieving all that. Let us get started on these amazing recipes.

Juicing Recipes For Weight Loss

Juicing is one of the fastest, natural and healthy ways you can lose weight. Juicing keeps your energy level high at all times, prevents hunger so you eat less snacks, its natural and limits your exposure to processed foods, provides a tasty way to eating raw vegetables, and helps detox your body after unhealthy diet choices. When you incorporate juicing in your weight loss program, you will be sure to get desired results.

There are two ways of juicing for weight loss; juice fasting and casual juicing. Juice fasting involves taking juices without solids for some time while casual juicing is when you include juices in your meal plan. For instance, you are replacing some meals with juice. Vegetable juices are better and healthier than fruit juices and are best for juicing to achieve weight loss, because vegetables contain less sugar than fruits. If you don't like the taste of vegetable juices, you can simply, add fruit or natural spices.

These great juicing recipes will help you achieve your weight loss goals.

Heart Beet

Ingredients

2 stalks of rainbow chard (silver beet)

2 green apples

1 broccoli stem

1 ½ beet with greens

1 lemon

2 stalks celery

1 large handful or parsley or basil

Instructions

Peel the lemon and beet. Wash all ingredients and put them in a juicer. Process and enjoy!

Calories 408; Protein 22.1 g; Sugar 36.6 g; Cholesterol 0 mg.

Mean Green

Ingredients

6 kale leaves

2 medium apples

1 tablespoon ginger

4 large stalks of celery

1 cucumber

½ lemon

Instructions

Wash all the products then process all ingredients in a juicer, then stir or shake and serve.

Calories 314; Protein 11g; Sugar 33.6g; Cholesterol 0 mg.

Don't Forget your Roots

Ingredients

1 sweet potato

1 beet root

10 medium carrots

Instructions

Put the ingredients in a juicer in the order; beet followed by sweet potato, then lastly carrots.

Calories 421; Protein 9.5 g; Sugar 33.5 g; Cholesterol 0 mg.

Cucumber and Tomato Juice

Ingredients

3 ½ chopped tomatoes

¼ teaspoon cayenne pepper

½ teaspoon sea salt

1 stalk celery

Mint leaves

½ teaspoon ground black pepper

2 cups chopped cucumbers

Instructions

Put the cut vegetables in a juicer and process then add sea salt, ground black pepper and cayenne pepper. You can add few drops of stevia for sweetness. Pour the juice in a glass and garnish it with mint leaves. This juice is great for summer.

Calories 180; Protein 8.3 g; Sugar 0 g; Cholesterol 0 mg.

Carrot and Watercress Juice

Ingredients

1 chopped watercress

2-3 medium carrots

2 roma tomatoes diced

1 teaspoon of ground black pepper

½ cup of spinach

1 teaspoon of kosher salt

½ cup of cilantro

Instructions

Wash, peel then dice the carrots to small chunks that can fit into the juicer. Chop the rest of the vegetables. Put all the vegetables in a juicer and process. Pour the juice into a glass, garnish it with cilantro and enjoy.

Calories 130; Protein 4.4 g; Sugar 10.1g; Cholesterol 0 mg.

Celery and Beet juice

Ingredients

1 small beet, cubed

4-5 celery stalks

1 cup coarsely chopped spinach

1 bunch cilantro

1 teaspoon sea salt

A little lemon juice

Instructions

Put all the ingredients in a juicer and process. Pour the juice in a glass and add lemon for flavor.

Calories 97.5; Protein 4.6g; Sugar 6.5 g; Cholesterol 0 mg.

Splendid Spinach

Ingredients

1 cup spinach

2 kale leaves

2 medium Apples

1 handful Parsley

Instructions

Process all ingredients in juicer jar at high, stir and serve in glass.

Calories 220; Protein 6.3 g; Sugar 32.2 g; Cholesterol 0 mg.

Apple and Spinach Juice

Ingredients

2 cups coarsely chopped spinach

2 medium apples, cubed

1 teaspoon kosher salt

¼ teaspoon cayenne pepper

½ cup red lettuce leaves or carrot greens

A little lemon juice

Instructions

Put all the ingredients in a juicer and process. Pour into a glass and enjoy.

Calories 155; Protein 1.4 g; Sugar 29.2 g; Cholesterol 0 mg.

Rainbow Blitz

Ingredients

5 medium carrots

1 thumb ginger root

1 cucumber

1 medium Apple

1 lemon

1 medium pear

2 handfuls spinach

Instructions

Process all ingredients in a juicer, stir or shake and serve.

Calories 419; Protein 9.6 g; Sugar 45 g; Cholesterol 0 mg.

Lemon and Watermelon Juice

Ingredients

1 cup watermelon with seeds

1 lemon

1 teaspoon mint leaves

Directions

Put all the ingredients in a juicer jar and process.

Calories 60; Protein 13.2 g; Sugar 11.1 g; Cholesterol 0 mg.

Tasty Green

Ingredients

1 cucumber

1 large orange (peeled and deseeded)

2 medium apples

6 kale leaves

4 stalks large celery

1 thumb of ginger root

½ lemon

Instructions

Process all ingredients in a juicer, stir or shake and serve.

Calories 372; Protein 11 g; Sugar45.5 g; Cholesterol 0 mg.

Juicing Recipes For Improved Immunity

Your immune system is comprised of organs, cells, and tissues whose sole purpose is to keep you healthy. Without it, your body would succumb to the bacteria, viruses and fungus all around us. To keep your immune system functioning, your body needs all the vitamins and minerals present in plants. Our bodies are a careful balance of good and bad bacteria and viruses. Antibiotics and pesticides kill both the good and bad bacterium in our guts and bodies. Up to 80% of our immune system is in our guts, so it is important to take proper care of it.

When our immune system functions properly, it identifies and destroys any threats to our body's systems and its organs. If the immune system is not working properly, or is overworked, it can miss or not be able to attack the invaders, allowing illness and infection. When our system is out of balance, it creates inflammation. Inflammation is any swelling or pain felt in the body. This is a signal that there is an underlying issue, and your immune system could use some support.

Always listen to your body. If a recipe calls for a fruit or vegetable that makes you feel nauseous or sluggish, trade it for an item which your body craves. All of our bodies work differently, and what might be energizing for me, may be a vitamin which your body does not need or does not utilize well. Keeping a food and juice diary and evaluating your mood, energy levels, and overall health during the first few weeks of incorporating juicing, or any other lifestyle or diet change, will help you pin down what is working, and what is not.

The right combination of vegetables and fruits contains all the essential nutrients that your body needs for improved immunity. Let us look at some of these recipes for an improved immunity.

Immune-Boosting Grapefruit juice

Ingredients

1 beet

1 pomelo grapefruit

2 celery stalks

½ inch (2.5 cm) piece of turmeric

2 carrots

½ inch (2.5 cm) piece of ginger

1 lemon

Instructions

Wash all produce well. Peel the beet, lemon and grapefruit. Put all the ingredients in a juicer, process and enjoy.

Calories 188; Protein 4.5 g; Sugar 29.5 g; Cholesterol 0 mg.

Red Tangy Juice

Ingredients

1 beet root

5 large carrots

2 large celery stalks

1 thumb ginger root

½ lime

1 pepper (jalapeno)

2 cups spinach

Instructions

Process all the ingredients in a juicer and serve. You should de-seed the jalapeno before juicing it if you don't want your juice to be too hot.

Calories 205; Protein 7.3 g; Sugar 20.6 g; Cholesterol 0 mg.

The Brain Stimulator juice

Ingredients

1 sweet potato

1 hard pear

1 grape fruit

1 orange

Instructions

Peel the orange and grape and try to keep as much of the white pith on them. Keep the sweet potato peel. Process in juicer and serve your juice.

Calories 352; Protein 5.2 g; Sugar 43.2 g; Cholesterol 0 mg.

Golden Juice

Ingredients

3 large carrots

4 large celery stalks

1 golden beet root

½ cucumber

1 medium pear (bosc)

½ thumb ginger root

Instructions

Process all the ingredients in a juicer, shake or stir and serve.

Calories 238; Protein 5.5 g; Sugar 29.2 g; Cholesterol 0 mg.

Immunity-Booster Juice

Ingredients

1 lemon

1 inch slice of ginger

3 medium carrots

4 stalks of celery

4 kiwi fruit

A handful of parsley

Instructions

Process all ingredients in juicer and serve.

Calories 338; Protein 7.9 g; Sugar 11.3 g; Cholesterol 0 mg.

Turmeric Sunrise

Ingredients

3 medium carrots

3 large celery stalks

2 medium apples

2 medium pears

1 thumb ginger root

2 Lemons, peeled

6 thumb turmeric root

Instructions

Process all ingredients in a juicer jar, shake well or stir and serve.

Calories 523; Protein 7.3 g; Sugar 68.9 g; Cholesterol mg.

The Minty Beta

Ingredients

4 carrots

Small handful of diced mint leaves

½ teaspoon spirulina

Instructions

Process all ingredients in juicer and serve.

Calories 118; Protein 14.9 g; Sugar 13.2 g; Cholesterol 0 mg.

Green Citrus

Ingredients

3 large celery stalks

1 sweet potato

2 medium apples

1 orange, peeled

2 medium pears

Instructions

Process all ingredients in a juicer, stir or shake and serve.

Calories 533; Protein 6.5 g; Sugar 68.5 g; Cholesterol 0 mg.

Sweet N Tart Citrus

Ingredients

2 oranges

2 medium apples

1 cup, whole cranberries

½ small grapefruit, peeled

1 teaspoon honey

½ lime

1 thumb ginger root

1 cup pineapple chunks

Instructions

Process all ingredients in a juicer, shake or stir and serve.

Calories 383; Protein 4.4 g; Sugar 72.2 g; Cholesterol 0 mg.

Immune Booster

Ingredients

1 piece of turmeric root

1 piece of ginger root

1 cup of parsley

1 cup of cilantro

5 carrots

Instructions

Juice the parsley and cilantro, followed by the turmeric and ginger root, and finally the carrots. Stir or shake and serve.

Calories 278; Protein 7.9 g; Sugar 15.9 g; Cholesterol 0 mg.

Morning Coffee

Ingredients

1 teaspoon ground cayenne pepper

4 cloves of garlic

½ cup of apple cider vinegar

1 cup of filtered water

Instructions

Warm the filtered water, and chop or grind the garlic. Add the apple cider vinegar, cayenne pepper, and garlic to the water. Stir and enjoy.

Calories 23.6; Protein 1 g; Sugar .3 g; Cholesterol 0 mg.

Garlic Tonic

Ingredients

5 cloves of garlic

1 cup of parsley

2 slices of lemon

1 cup of filtered water

Instructions

Juice the garlic, parsley and lemon, and add to a cup of filtered water. Stir and enjoy.

Calories 55; Protein 2.8 g; Sugar 2.1 g; Cholesterol 0 mg.

Cold Tonic

Ingredients

1 cup of organic bone or chicken broth

1 cup of parsley

2 carrots

2 celery stalks

½ onion

Instructions

Juice the parsley, celery, onion, and carrots. Pour juice into cup of warm or room temperature bone broth. Stir and enjoy.

Calories 102; Protein 4.9 g; Sugar 7.1 g; Cholesterol 0 mg.

Cough Buster

Ingredients

2 cups of pineapple

2 carrots

1 cup of spinach

Instructions

Juice the pineapple, followed by the spinach and carrots. Stir or shake and serve.

Calories 209; Protein 3.3 g; Sugar 37.7 g; Cholesterol 0 mg.

Juicing Recipes For Detox

It's important to keep the liver and the kidney free from toxins. These detox recipes are essential to boost your body cleansing mechanism. Beets are great for liver cleansing, cranberries are good for the bladder, ginger, lemons and apples cleanse the entire body, greens nourish and clean our cells, dandelion leaves are great for the liver, cucumber and celery are natural diuretics.

The following juices are highly effective for detox.

Radiant Orange Juice

Ingredients

3 carrots

2 small oranges

1 – 2 cucumbers

1 inch (2.5 cm) piece of ginger

1 yellow bell pepper (capsicum)

Instructions

Wash all produce well. Cut carrots and cucumbers and peel oranges. Process all ingredients in a juicer and enjoy.

Calories 300; Protein 9.1 g; Sugar 33.4g; Cholesterol 0 mg.

The Detox juice

Ingredients

1 handful of spinach

2 apples

¼ cucumber

1 handful of mixed green leaves like parsley and watercress

1 stick of celery

Ice cubes

Instructions

Process all the ingredients in a juicer and serve.

Calories 199; Protein 5.2 g; Sugar 29.5 g; Cholesterol 0 mg.

Great Green Juice

Ingredients

½ cucumber

3 large celery stalks

3 medium whole tomatoes

½ medium pepper (sweet green)

2 handfuls parsley

1 cup spinach

2 large carrots

Instructions

Process all the ingredients in a juicer jar, shake well or stir then serve.

Calories 242; Protein 9.8 g; Sugar 12.2 g; Cholesterol 0 mg.

Kidney Cleansing Juice

Ingredients

1 ounce of parsley

1 apple

3 stalks of celery

1 large cucumber

3 medium to large carrots

1 inch ginger

Instructions

Put all the ingredients in a juicer processing then serve as desired

Calories 247; Protein 9.2 g; Sugar 20.9 g; Cholesterol 0 mg.

Veggie Blueberry

Ingredients

1 stalk broccoli

6 large carrots

1 medium apple (granny smith)

1 cup blueberry

1 medium whole tomato

Directions

Put all ingredients in a juicer, process, and stir or shake well then serve.

Calories 398; Protein 11.1 g; Sugar 49.2 g; Cholesterol 0 mg.

Holiday Lemonade

Ingredients

3 medium apples

½ cup whole cranberries

¼ thumb ginger root

½ fruit lemon

1 large orange

Directions

Put all ingredients in a juicer, process, shake or stir then serve.

Calories 311; Protein 2.6 g; Sugar 58.4 g; Cholesterol 0 mg.

Turmeric Sunrise

Ingredients

1 thumb ginger root

3 large celery stalks

3 medium carrots

2 medium apples

2 lemons (peeled)

2 medium pears

6 thumb turmeric root

Directions

Process all the ingredients in a juicer then shake or stir and serve.

Calories 442; Protein 5.5 g; Sugar 66.8 g; Cholesterol 0 mg.

Berry Juice

Ingredients

3 cups strawberries

½ lime

2 large apples

Instructions

Process all ingredients in a juicer, shake or stir and serve.

Calories 378; Protein 5.5 g; Sugar 63.3 g; Cholesterol 0 mg.

Hangover Juice

This juice is rich in protein and great for hangovers. Drink plenty of water for this juice to work best

Ingredients

2 large celery stalks

1 teaspoon Spirulina (dried)

3 cups spinach

1 beet root

Instructions

Put all the ingredients in a juicer, process, shake well or stir then serve.

Calories 77; Protein 4.9g; Sugar 5.9g; Cholesterol 0 mg.

Beets Juice

Ingredients

3 medium carrots

1 beet root

½ lemon

2 leaves of red cabbage

¼ Pineapples

1 orange

2 handfuls spinach

Instructions

Put all ingredients in a juicer, process, shake or stir and serve.

Calories 265; Protein 7.3 g; Sugar 41.3 g; Cholesterol 0 mg.

The Liver Cleanser

Ingredients

4 medium carrots

1 beet root

3 leaves beet greens

1 large celery stalk

1 large apple

½ thumb Ginger Root

Instructions

Put all ingredients in a juicer, process, shake or stir then serve.

Calories 228; Protein 6.2 g; Sugar 31.6 g; Cholesterol 0 mg.

Vegetable Detox Juice

Ingredients

1 tomato

3 spears of asparagus

1 cup of lettuce

2 carrots

Instructions

Wash the vegetables then process in a juicer. You can add Splenda and some lemon to add some flavor. Pour in a glass and enjoy.

Calories 95; Protein 4.2 g; Sugar 5.6 g; Cholesterol 0 mg.

Super Detox Juice

Ingredients

1 beet

2 Carrots

1 cucumber

1 stalk of celery

Instructions

Process in a juicer and enjoy.

Calories 134; Protein 5.1g; Sugar 11.1 g; Cholesterol 0 mg.

Antioxidant Juice

Ingredients

1 apple

½ small onion

1 broccoli head

3 stalks of celery

1 clove of garlic

Instructions

Process all the ingredients in juicer, serve and enjoy.

Calories 298; Protein 20.7 g; Sugar 14.4 g; Cholesterol 0 mg.

Beet Blackberry Juice

Ingredients

2-3 apples

3 small beets

½ inch fresh ginger

8 ounces blackberries

Instructions

Process ingredients in juicer then serve.

Calories 403; Protein 6.1 g; Sugar 69.8 g; Cholesterol 0 mg.

Detoxifying Juice

This fruit juice is tremendous for liver cleansing:

Ingredients

2 avocados

2 apples

Instructions

Process ingredients in a juicer and enjoy.

Calories 793; Protein 7.8 g; Sugar 44.1 g; Cholesterol 0 mg.

Alkaline Liver Cleanse

Ingredients

1 clove grated garlic

1 inch grated ginger

2 lemons

1 grapefruit

1 tablespoon of flax oil

1 tablespoon of acidophilus

Instructions

Wash and peel the grapefruit and lemon if not organic. Put all the ingredients in a juicer and process until ready. Serve and enjoy.

Calories 220; Protein 2.1 g; Sugar 20.1 g; Cholesterol 0 mg.

Liver Detox

Ingredients

2 stalks of celery

1 small cabbage

2 pears

1 cup of watercress

Instructions

Wash and peel the pear. Cut the cabbage in pieces. Process all the ingredients in a juicer and serve.

Calories 363; Protein 13 g; Sugar 27.4 g; Cholesterol 0 mg.

Golden Carrot Orange juice

Carrot juice is full of vitamins B and E, beta-carotene and a variety of minerals. Orange has vitamin C while golden beets are rich in calcium and potassium.

Ingredients

3 cara cara navels

2 golden beets

½ inch of fresh ginger

4 carrots

Instructions

Wash, peel and cut carrots and beet. Put in the juicer jar add the navels and the ginger the process until ready then serve.

Calories 213; Protein 5.8 g; Sugar 32 g; Cholesterol 0 mg.

Cleansing Juice

Ingredients

½ beets with greens

3 carrots

½ cucumber or ½ zucchini

Instructions

Chop the carrots, cucumber and beets then process all the ingredients in a juicer then serve the juice.

Calories 127; Protein 3.4 g; Sugar 19.8 g; Cholesterol 0 mg.

High Antioxidant Juice

Ingredients

1 stalk of celery

1 cucumber

2 large tomatoes

3-5 grinds of fresh ground black pepper

½ teaspoon sea salt

½ red bell pepper

1-3 shakes cayenne pepper

Instructions

Cut the tomatoes into quarters, slice the cucumber and add to juicer then add pepper and salt. Process and then enjoy.

Calories 112; Protein 4.6 g; Sugar 3 g; Cholesterol 0 mg.

Juicing Recipes For Strong Bones And Teeth

The following juices contain all the important nutrients for strong bones and teeth. These juices contain high amounts calcium and other essential nutrients to help protect your bones from degeneration.

Bone Health Juice

Ingredients

½ apple

6 carrots

4 sprigs of parsley

4 kale leaves

Instructions

Wash all the ingredients and process them in a juicer. Serve in a glass and enjoy.

Calories 299; Protein 11.5 g; Sugar 29 g; Cholesterol 0 mg.

High Potassium Drink

Ingredients

1 apple

3 large carrots

2 stalks of celery

Handful of fresh spinach

Handful of fresh parsley

½ lemon, peeled

Instructions

Prepare and process the ingredients in a juicer then serve.

Calories 204; Protein 4.8 g; Sugar 25.2 g; Cholesterol 0 mg.

Beach Juice

Ingredients

Small handful of parsley

3-4 tangerines

1 1-inch thick pineapple round

Instructions

Peel the tangerines. Add all the ingredients to a juicer, process then serve.

Calories 269; Protein 4.7 g; Sugar 53.8 g; Cholesterol 0 mg.

Muscle Juice

Ingredients

1 bunch of spinach

2 medium apples

½ lemon, peeled

Instructions

Peel the lemon. Process all the ingredients in a juicer then serve.

Calories 165; Protein 2.5 g; Sugar 29.7 g; Cholesterol 0 mg.

Healthy Bones Juice

Ingredients

2 large carrots

1 apple

½ cup fresh broccoli

½ lemon

1 small handful of parsley, fresh and organic

Instructions

Peel the lemon. Process all the ingredients in juicer and then add 1 teaspoon of agave nectar to the juice. Enjoy the drink.

Calories 149; Protein 3.2 g; Sugar 20.6 g; Cholesterol 0 mg.

Lettuce Juice

Ingredients

4 large romaine lettuce leaves

3 large carrots

6 spinach leaves

4 sprigs of parsley

¼ large turnip

Instructions

Add all the ingredients to the juicer and process. Stir or shake and serve.

Calories 120; Protein 5 g; Sugar 11.6 g; Cholesterol 0 mg.

Strawberry Pineapple Juice

Ingredients

1 orange

5 strawberries

2 1-inch pineapple rounds

Instructions

Peel the oranges. Add all the ingredients to the juicer and process. Stir or shake and serve.

Calories 185; Protein 2.6 g; Sugar 36.8 g; Cholesterol 0 mg.

Cucumber and Celery Juice

Ingredients

1 cucumber

1 ½ stalks of celery

2 large apples

Instructions

Add all the ingredients to the juicer and process. Serve as desired

Calories 275; Protein 3.8 g; Sugar 44.1 g; Cholesterol 0 mg.

High Iron Juice

This is a great juice for healthy bones

Ingredients

1 apple

¼ pineapple

¼ banana

1 cup natural yoghurt (soya if vegan)

½ teaspoon spirulina

Instructions

Process all the ingredients in a juicer, process and serve.

Calories 311; 14 Protein g; 47.4 Sugar g; Cholesterol 0 mg.

Healthy Bones Cocktail

Kale and parsley are loaded with boron, magnesium, and vitamin and other minerals vital for healthy bones.

Ingredients

1 large kale leaf

1 celery stalk

1 handful parsley

1 lemon

1 cucumber

1-inch chunk ginger root

Instructions

Peel the lemon and the cucumber if not organic, scrub and peel ginger if old. Cut produce to fit your juicer's feed tube. Juice ingredients and stir. Pour into a glass and enjoy.

Calories 93; Protein 4.8 g; Sugar 6 g; Cholesterol 0 mg.

Juicing Recipes For Healthy Skin

Juicing fresh fruits and vegetables has a long-term tremendous effect on your skin tone and texture. Preparing fruits and vegetables in the right combination for juicing detoxifies the liver, which means that it gets rid of all the toxins in your blood and tissues, restores alkalinity, and balances your body system.

Use the following juicing recipes for healthy and radiant skin. The fruits and vegetables incorporated contain high amounts of potassium, magnesium, silica and all the essential nutrients for good complexion, radiant and youthful skin

Sweet Skin Juice

Ingredients

2 kale leaves

6 carrots

1 apple

Instructions

Chop carrot, apple and kale. Process and serve.

Calories 295; Protein 9 g; Sugar 34.4 g; Cholesterol 0 mg.

Cucumber Wrinkle Reducer Juice

Ingredients

1 large cucumber

2 apples

1 celery stalk

2 carrots

Instructions

Process the ingredients in a juicer then serve.

Calories 243; Protein 4.4 g; Sugar 34.3 g; Cholesterol 0 mg.

Skin Soothing Juice

Ingredients

1 cucumber

8 carrots

½ bunch of Spinach

Instructions

Wash the vegetables then chop spinach, carrots and cucumber. Process the ingredients and serve.

Calories 253; Protein 8.6 g; Sugar 22.7 g; Cholesterol 0 mg.

Smooth Skin Juice

This juice helps fight psoriasis, eczema, and rosacea

Ingredients

¼ medium-sized cucumber

½ bulb fennel

1 large apple

1 large carrot

½ ripe avocados

Instructions

Process the fennel, apple, carrot and cucumber in a juicer then transfer the mixed juice to a blender. Add the avocado flesh and then process until smooth then serve.

Calories 432; Protein 6.3 g; Sugar 17.7 g; Cholesterol 0 mg.

Smooth Perfecter Juice

This is a great juice for dry and mature skin.

Ingredients

2 large apples or 200ml fresh apple juice

Handful (about 30) blackberries, blueberries, or pitted dark cherries

Handful (about 30) seedless black grapes

½ tablespoon cold-pressed flaxseed walnut, rapeseed, or olive oil

Instructions

Process the apples, transfer to a blender with the grapes and your choice of, blackberries, blueberries or cherries. Blend until smooth. Stir in your choice of plant oil before serving.

Calories 390; Protein 2.2 g; Sugar 53.7 g; Cholesterol 0 mg.

Tomato Orange Age Restorer Recipe

Tomatoes have antioxidant lycopene, which has anti-aging properties.

Ingredients

2 oranges

2 celery stalks

1 apple

5 ripe tomatoes

Small slice of ginger root

Instructions

Process all ingredients in juicer and serve as desired.

Calories 274; Protein 8.6 g; Sugar 24.8 g; Cholesterol 0 mg.

Greenie Genie

This juice is the perfect remedy for clearing acne, blemishes and other skin problems

Ingredients

4 small asparagus spears

2 medium carrots

2 cm cube ginger, unpeeled

2 medium apples

Small handful freshly cut wheatgrass, or 1 teaspoon of powdered greens, like spirulina, chlorella or wheatgrass

Small handful parsley

Instructions

Process all the ingredients in a juicer, stir in the powdered greens (if using). Serve in a glass and enjoy.

Calories 224; Protein 11.6 g; Sugar 32.4 g; Cholesterol 0 mg.

Cucumber Apple Juice

This juice is loaded with silicon and other hydrating minerals and vitamins, which nourish your skin.

Ingredients

1 cucumber

½ lemon

2 stalks celery

1 inch ginger

1 apple

Instructions

Wash all vegetables and fruits. You can leave unpeeled if organic. Peel lightly if inorganic. Put ingredients into a juicer and process in the order; cucumber first, followed by the apple, ginger, lemon and finally the celery. Pour over ice for a cooled juice and enjoy.

Calories 126; Protein 2.5 g; Sugar 17.9 g; Cholesterol 0 mg.

Tropical Dream Juice

Ingredients

4 cups papaya

9 ½ cups carrots

Instructions

Chop carrots and papaya the process in juicer and serve.

Calories 456; Protein 9.1 g; Sugar 59.6 g; Cholesterol 0 mg.

Wrinkle Free Juice

Ingredients

2 cucumbers

1 1-inch knob of ginger root

2 medium oranges

Instructions

Peel the oranges leaving as much of the white pith inside the skin. Process in a juicer then serve and enjoy.

Calories 204; Protein 2.6 g; Sugar 24.9 g; Cholesterol 0 mg.

Juicing Recipes for Health Hair & Nails

Like your skin, your hair and nails require loads of vitamin A, as well as B vitamins to stay in top shape. The health of your hair and nails can tell a lot about your overall health. Let's review some of the best juices if you are struggling with damaged hair or brittle nails.

Orange Splash

Ingredients

2 medium carrots

1 cup diced butternut squash

2 medium peaches

1 peeled orange

Instructions

Peel oranges, and then process in this order: oranges, peaches, squash, then carrots. Stir or shake and serve.

Calories 340; Protein 6.8 g; Sugar 48.5 g; Cholesterol 0 mg.

Beauty is Root Deep

Ingredients

1 cup diced butternut squash

2 medium carrots

1 cup diced pumpkin

1 tsp of cinnamon

Instructions

Process the carrots, squash and pumpkin, then add the cinnamon to taste. Stir or shake and serve.

Calories 215; Protein 5.7 g; Sugar 13.7 g; Cholesterol 0 mg.

Berry Blast

Ingredients

1 cup of whole strawberries

1 cup of raspberries

1 cup of blueberries

1 medium apple

Instructions

Dice the apples to process easier and rinse the berries well. Process the berries followed by the apples, then stir or shake and serve.

Calories 241; Protein 7.1 g; Sugar 22.4 g; Cholesterol 0 mg.

Pineapple Kale Refresh

Ingredients

2 green apples

2 cups diced pineapple

2 cups of kale

Instructions

Dice the apples and pineapple to process easier. Process the kale, then the pineapple, and finally the apple. Stir or shake and serve.

Calories 384; Protein 6.1 g; Sugar 69.3 g; Cholesterol 0 mg.

Tomato Greens Juice

Ingredients

2 medium tomatoes or 2 cups of baby tomatoes

2 cups of spinach

2 cloves of garlic

Instructions

Juice the spinach followed by the tomatoes, and finally the garlic. Stir or shake and serve.

Calories 137; Protein 2.6 g; Sugar 23.2 g; Cholesterol 0 mg.

Hair-Thickening Juice

Ingredients

1 medium carrot

1 cup alfalfa sprouts

1 cabbage leaves or 2 Brussels sprouts

1 medium beet & beet greens

1 cup broccoli florets

½ -1 clove Garlic (optional)

2 slices red onion

Instructions

Wash all ingredients then process in your juicer. Add apples and or watermelon to get a sweet taste. Serve and enjoy.

Calories 154; Protein 9.7 g; Sugar 8.5 g; Cholesterol 0 mg.

Hair Growth Tonic

Ingredients

1 cucumber

1 cup of alfalfa sprouts

1 cup of spinach

1 lemon

1 large carrot or two medium carrots

2 apples

2 stalks of celery

1 inch piece of ginger

Instructions

Chop carrots, peel lemon and then process all the ingredients in a juicer. Stir or shake and serve.

Calories 239; Protein 5.7 g; Sugar 35.2 g; Cholesterol 0 mg.

Juicing Recipes For Good Eyesight

The fruits and vegetable used in the following juicing recipes for good eyesight are rich in vitamin A and other essential nutrients.

Peachy Keen

Ingredients

½ lemon

5 medium peaches

3 tablespoons fresh basil

14 medium carrots

Directions

Juice in this order for best flavor: start with the basil, then lemon followed by peaches and finally carrots. Serve the juice.

Calories 571; Protein 12.2 g; Sugar 85.2 g; Cholesterol 0 mg.

The Eye Opener

Ingredients

14 medium carrots

2 medium apples

2 small oranges

Directions

Peel oranges then process all ingredients in a juicer, shake or stir and serve.

Calories 617; Protein 11.5 g; Sugar 92.7 g; Cholesterol mg.

Peach Medley

Ingredients

½ lemon

10 medium carrots

1 large orange

2 large apples

2 large peaches

Instructions

Peel the lemon and oranges then process all ingredients in a juicer, shake well or stir and serve.

Calories 547; Protein 9.4 g; Sugar 87.9 g; Cholesterol 0 mg.

Lemon Essence

Ingredients

8 medium carrots

1 medium apple

1 thumb ginger root

1 fruit lemon

Instructions

Process all ingredients in a juicer, stir or shake and serve.

Calories 282; Protein5.3 g; Sugar 37.6 g; Cholesterol 0 mg.

Juicing Recipes For General Health

There are tremendous health benefits in consuming one glass of raw vegetable juice every day. For instance, juicing provides a fast and efficient way for our bodies to absorb essential nutrients. The following recipes will ensure you live a healthy long life.

Hair-Thickening Juice

Ingredients

1 medium carrot

1 cup alfalfa sprouts

1 cabbage leaves or 2 Brussels sprouts

1 medium beet & beet greens

1 cup broccoli florets

½ -1 clove Garlic (optional)

2 slices red onion

Instructions

Wash all ingredients then process in your juicer. Add apples and or watermelon to get a sweet taste. Serve and enjoy.

Calories 154; Protein 9.7 g; Sugar 8.5 g; Cholesterol 0 mg

Hair Growth Tonic

Ingredients

1 cucumber

1 cup of alfalfa sprouts

1 cup of spinach

1 lemon

1 large carrot or two medium carrots

2 apples

2 stalks of celery

1 inch piece of ginger

Instructions

Chop carrots, peel lemon and then process all the ingredients in a juicer then serve.

Calories 239; Protein 5.7 g; Sugar 35.2 g; Cholesterol 0 mg.

The Cancer Killer

Ingredients

1 celery stalk

1 carrot

½ potato

1 beet

1 radish

Instructions

Cut potato, carrot and beet into small pieces. Process all ingredients in a juicer, serve and enjoy.

Calories 150; Protein 3.9 g; Sugar 14.1 g; Cholesterol 0 mg.

Workout and Recovery Juice

This juice is high in potassium and sodium essential nutrients for working out.

Ingredients

1 stick celery

¼ small cucumber

2 apples

Ice

Instructions

Juice all the ingredients and pour over ice. Put it in a flask and enjoy 1 hour after working out or 30 minutes before.

Calories 164; Protein 1.7 g; Sugar 28.7 g; Cholesterol 0 mg.

Parsley Energy Juice

Ingredients

1 apple

2 carrots

1 stalk celery

1 large bunch of parsley

Instructions

A centrifugal juicer is recommended. To get the best results, process parsley with carrots or celery first then add the apple last. Serve and enjoy.

Calories 135; Protein 2.2 g; Sugar 20 g; Cholesterol 0 mg.

Energizing Juice

Ingredients

1 organic cucumber

4 leaf organic lacinato kale

5 stalks organic celery

3 cups organic spinach

½ bunch organic parsley

Instructions

Process all the ingredients in a juicer. Add either a small organic green apple or an organic beet to add a sweet flavor if it's not sweet enough then serve and enjoy.

Calories 150; Protein 2.1 g; Sugar 9.7 g; Cholesterol 0 mg.

Beet Energizer juice

Ingredients

2 medium carrots

1 large apple

1 medium beetroot

Sprig of fresh mint, leaves only

3cm (1¼in) cube ginger, unpeeled

Slice of lemon, to serve (optional)

Instructions

Juice all the ingredients in your juicer. When placing ingredients in juicer, sandwich herbs or leaves between chunks of apple, carrot or beetroot. This helps flush them through the juicer. Serve with a slice of lemon.

Calories 180; Protein 3.7 g; Sugar 29.1 g; Cholesterol 0 mg.

Carrot, Tomato and Cucumber Juice

This juice helps in lowering blood sugar thus good for diabetics.

Ingredients

1 carrot

2 ripe tomatoes

1 cucumber

Instructions

Process all the ingredients in a juicer then serve and enjoy.

Calories 116; Protein 4.8 g; Sugar 2.8 g; Cholesterol 0 mg.

Cancer Prevention Healthy Heart Juice

Ingredients

3 stalks of celery

3 medium tomatoes

4 kale leaves

2 medium to large carrots

Instructions

Put all the ingredients in a juicer. Process and serve.

Calories 231; Protein 8.8 g; Sugar 10.7 g; Cholesterol mg.

Juicing Recipes for Energy

Low energy is one of the most common health complaints. Between the stress of our busy lives, lack of sleep, and our low fruit and vegetable diet, the average person simply does not have enough energy. Juicing can improve your energy levels by providing the necessary vitamins and minerals required by your body to thrive. It can also aid in detoxification and help your body rid itself of toxins slowing it down. Finally, juicing can help your organs function properly, digesting food quickly and fully while pulling out the essential vitamins and minerals. Most find that after a few weeks of juicing, and especially after a juice cleanse, that their energy has dramatically improved. Try these recipes to bring more energy into your everyday life!

Parsley Energy Juice

Ingredients

1 apple

2 carrots

1 stalk celery

1 large bunch of parsley

Instructions

A centrifugal juicer is recommended. To get the best results, process parsley with carrots or celery first then add the apple last. Serve and enjoy.

Calories 135; Protein 2.2 g; Sugar 20.0 g; Cholesterol 0 mg.

Energizing Juice

Ingredients

1 organic cucumber

4 leaf organic lacinato kale

5 stalks organic celery

3 cups organic spinach

½ bunch organic parsley

Instructions

Process all the ingredients in a juicer. Add either a small organic green apple or an organic beet to add a sweet flavor if it's not sweet enough then serve and enjoy.

Calories 95; Protein 6.9 g; Sugar 4.8 g; Cholesterol 0 mg.

Beet Energizer juice

Ingredients

2 medium carrots

1 large apple

1 medium beetroot

Sprig of fresh mint, leaves only

3cm (1¼in) cube ginger, unpeeled

Slice of lemon, to serve (optional)

Instructions

Juice all the ingredients in your juicer. When placing ingredients in juicer, sandwich herbs or leaves between chunks of apple, carrot or beetroot. This helps flush them through the juicer. Serve with a slice of lemon.

Calories 135; Protein 2.6 g; Sugar 20.7 g; Cholesterol 0 mg.

Afternoon Pick-Me-Up

Ingredients

1 organic green apple

4 cups of organic spinach

2 sweet potatoes

2 oranges

Instructions

Dice the apple and sweet potatoes to process easier, and peel the oranges. Juice the spinach, then the apple and potatoes, and finally the oranges. Stir or shake and serve.

Calories 282; Protein 8.7 g; Sugar 39.4 g; Cholesterol 0 mg.

Citrus Burst

Ingredients

2 oranges

1 grapefruit

2 organic green apples

5 medium carrots

Instructions

Peel the oranges and grapefruit, and cut up the apples, carrots, and grapefruit to process easier if desired. Process the oranges and grapefruit, followed by the apples and carrots. Stir or shake and serve.

Calories 466; Protein 7.5 g; Sugar 84.6 g; Cholesterol 0 mg.

Orange Energy Blast

Ingredients

2 oranges

5 medium carrots

1 sweet potatoes

Instructions

Peel the oranges, and dice the sweet potatoes and carrots. Process the oranges, followed by the sweet potatoes and carrots. Stir or shake, then serve.

Calories 385; Protein 7.5 g; Sugar 38.8 g; Cholesterol 0 mg.

Green Punch

Ingredients

2 cups of organic spinach

2 cups of organic arugula

1 cup of sprouts (broccoli or radish)

½ bunch of organic parsley

½ bunch of organic cilantro

2 organic green apples

Slice of lemon, to serve (optional)

Instructions

Rinse all of your greens, and juice these first. Then, dice and juice your apples. Garnish with a squeeze of lemon if desired. Stir or shake and serve.

Calories 126; Protein 5.8 g; Sugar 29.1 g; Cholesterol 0 mg.

Hawaiian Morning Juice

Ingredients

2 cups papaya

2 cups of pineapple

2 oranges

Slice of lemon, to serve (optional)

Instructions

Peel the oranges, and slice the pineapple and papaya. Juice the oranges, followed by the papaya and pineapple. Garnish with a squeeze of lemon, if desired. Stir or shake and serve.

Calories 385; Protein 5.3 g; Sugar 73.3 g; Cholesterol 0 mg.

Tropical Pineapple Juice

Ingredients

2 cups of pineapple

2 organic green apples

2 oranges

1 cup of organic strawberries

Slice of lemon, to serve (optional)

Instructions

Peel the oranges, and cut off the strawberry leaves if desired. Dice the pineapple and apples to process easier, if desired. Process the oranges, pineapple and strawberries, followed by the apples. Garnish with a squeeze of lemon if desired.

Calories 464; Protein 5.2 g; Sugar 93.5 g; Cholesterol 0 mg.

Cholesterol Lowering Juicing Recipes

The following recipes are effective in lowering cholesterol levels in your system.

Carrot Green Apple Juice

Ingredients

2 green apples

2 carrots

2 ribs celery or half a cucumber

Instructions

Process the ingredients in a juicer then serve.

Calories 214; Protein 2.8 g; Sugar 34.8 g; Cholesterol 0 mg.

Spinach Mixed Juice

Ingredients

2 carrots

3-4 kale leaves

2 green apples

1 cup of broccoli

Instructions

Wash the produce then process ingredients in juicer then serve.

Calories 188; Protein5.2 g; Sugar 2.8g; Cholesterol 0 mg.

Carrot Grape Juice

Ingredients

2 carrots

1 grapefruit

1 cup of grapes

Instructions

Chop the carrots then process all ingredients in juicer. Pour in a glass then serve.

Calories 187; Protein 3.1 g; Sugar 37.7 g; Cholesterol 0 mg.

Capsicum Apple Juice

Ingredients

2 ribs of celery

2 green apples

2 capsicums

1 slice of lemon (with peel)

Instructions

Process the ingredients in juicer then pour into a glass and enjoy.

Calories 173; Protein 3.7 g; Sugar 25.0 g; Cholesterol 0 mg.

Kale Green Apple Juice

Ingredients

1 cucumber

2 green apples

3-4 kale leaves

1 slice of lemon (with peel)

Instructions

Process all ingredients in your juicer then serve.

Calories 140; Protein 4.1 g; Sugar 19.5 g; Cholesterol 0 mg.

Cucuberry Juice

Ingredients

1 cup blueberries

1 cup strawberries

1 cup cranberries

1 cup raspberries

½ cucumber

Instructions

Put all ingredients in a juicer and process then serve as desired and enjoy.

Calories 246; Protein 3.8 g; Sugar 28.4 g; Cholesterol 0 mg.

Alkalizing Juice

Ingredients

1 organic cucumber

1 organic green apple

2 stalks organic celery

1 organic carrot

1 cup organic spinach

Instructions

Process all the ingredients in a juicer. You can omit the carrot if you are trying to maintain your sugar levels. Alternatively, you can still have carrot for a sweeter taste if necessary.

Calories 219; Protein 5.2 g; Sugar 28 g; Cholesterol 0 mg.

Carrot, Green Apple, Celery and Spinach juice

Ingredients

1 celery stalk

1 green apple

2 carrots

1 bunch of spinach

Instructions

Process all the ingredients in a juice jar then serve and enjoy.

Calories 246 ; Protein 6 g; Sugar 32 g; Cholesterol 0 mg.

Lean Green

Ingredients

2 Swiss chard leaves

1 orange

1 cucumber

2 medium apples

I thumb ginger root

1 lemon

30 peppermint leaves

Instructions

Process all ingredients in a juicer, shake or stir and serve.

Calories 290; Protein 7.4 g; Sugar43.8 g; Cholesterol 0 mg.

Healthy Heart Juice

Ingredients

2 organic tomatoes

1 handful organic parsley

6 sprigs organic watercress

2 organic green apples

Instructions

Process all the ingredients in a juice jar then serve.

Calories 201; Protein 3.4 g; Sugar 28.8 g; Cholesterol 0 mg.

Spicy Juice

Ingredients

1 orange

¼ fresh pineapple

½ handful cilantro

½ small jalapeno, seeded

Instructions

Process all the ingredients in a juicer and serve.

Calories 121; Protein 1.7 g; Sugar 24.7 g; Cholesterol 0 mg.

Bitter Gourd Juice

This juice is low in sugar and good in lowering your blood sugar levels.

Ingredients

½ bitter gourd

½ green apple

½ cucumber

½ capsicum (or green bell pepper)

2 celery stalks

Instructions

Process all the ingredients in a juice jar then serve.

Calories 104; Protein 3.0 g; Sugar 10.0 g; Cholesterol 0 mg.

Wild Spiced Berry Juice

Ingredients

1 cup dandelion leaves or more to taste

1 small chili with seeds and placental skin removed (optional)

2 cups strawberries

10-20 drops of alcohol-free liquid stevia (optional)

1 cup raspberries

Instructions

Process all the ingredients in a juicer and serve.

Calories 217; Protein 5.2 g; Sugar 16.0 g; Cholesterol 0 mg.

Broccoli Juice

This juice is effective in lowering blood sugar. This makes it a healthy juice for the diabetics.

Ingredients

3-4 carrots

1 stalk of broccoli

2 green apples

Instructions

Process all the ingredients in a juicer then serve.

Calories 286; Protein 7.6 g; Sugar 39.9 g; Cholesterol 0 mg.

Low Sugar Green Juice

Ingredients

3 kale leaves

2 handfuls of spinach

½ green apple

1 ½ cucumbers

3 limes, peeled

8 stems and leaves of mint

Directions

Wash all produce well. Peel limes or leave it unpeeled for zest. Juice all ingredients and serve.

Calories 210; Protein 10.4 g; Sugar 12.6 g; Cholesterol 0 mg.

Veggie Juice

Ingredients

1 cup organic spinach

2 stalks organic celery

1 medium organic red pepper

½ organic fennel bulb

½ bunch organic cilantro

½ organic cucumber

1 organic carrot

1 lime

Instructions

Process the ingredients in a juicer then squeeze more lime into the juice. You can add a clove of garlic, which works well in this juice.

Calories 118; Protein 5.3 g; Sugar 6.0 g; Cholesterol 0 mg.

Garden Green Juice

This juice is ideal for post work out

Ingredients

1 young Thai coconut

1 handful of spinach

1 handful of green kale

½ banana

Instructions

Crack open coconut carefully and then pour coconut water into your blender. Remove coconut meat with a spoon and add to blender. Add spinach and kale in juicer then process then transfer the juice to the blender, add the banana and process for 30 seconds, serve and enjoy.

Calories 237; Protein 5.3 g; Sugar 11.5 g; Cholesterol 0 mg.

Bountiful Health Juice

Ingredients

1 organic cucumber

2 cups organic string beans

10-12 organic Brussels sprouts

1 peeled organic lemon

Instructions

Process all ingredients in a juicer then serve.

Calories 152; Protein 5.2 g; Sugar 5.7 g; Cholesterol 0 mg.

The Ginger Juice

Ingredients

2 carrots

2 apples

¼ inch ginger

Ice cubes

1 slice of lemon

Instructions

Process all the ingredients in a juicer and serve.

Calories 204; Protein 2.1 g; Sugar 35.1 g; Cholesterol 0 mg.

Blossoming Juice

Ingredients

1 (2-inch) ginger

5 large Fuji apples, cored

1 medium lime

7 large sprigs cilantro sectioned

Instructions

Peel and slice fresh ginger, remove lime rind and process all the ingredients in a juicer. Serve and enjoy.

Calories 370; Protein 3.9 g; Sugar 72.6 g; Cholesterol 0 mg.

The Booster

This juice helps to control your blood pressure.

Ingredients

½ pineapple

2 apples

¼ cup alfalfa sprouts

¼ cup broccoli

¼ cup watercress

¼ cup parsley

¼ cup kale

1 teaspoon wheatgrass powder

Ice cubes

Instructions

Process all the ingredients in a juicer and serve.

Calories 315; Protein 3.6 g; Sugar 61.2 g; Cholesterol 0 mg.

Arthritis Soother

This juice helps soothe the aches & pains that arthritis sufferers endure. Use extra-virgin olive oil only; it is harmful to try and substitute with any other oil. You should also avoid dairy products while taking the juice to maximize benefits.

Ingredients

4 medium spear Asparagus

3 large celery stalks

1 broccoli stalk

3 large carrots

1 medium apple

1 tablespoon olive oil

1 handful parsley

Instructions

Process the ingredients in a juicer except the olive oil. Don't put olive oil into your juicer. Pour the olive oil into a glass, then empty the juice onto it and stir to mix well.

Calories 322; Protein 6.1 g; Sugar 22.8 g; Cholesterol 0 mg.

The Ultimate Green Juice

Ingredients

1 bunch celery

1 handful of flat leaf parsley leaves

1 lime

1 lemon

1 inch of fresh ginger

4-5 kale leaves

1 green apple

Instructions

Process all the ingredients in a juicer. Add one tablespoon of organic coconut oil for additional health benefits. Serve and enjoy.

Calories 174; Protein 4.6 g; Sugar 15.8 g; Cholesterol 0 mg.

Pineapple Juice

Ingredients

1 medium kiwi, peeled

1 (1-inch) peeled fresh ginger

1 small pineapple, peeled, cored, and sliced

½ cup fresh young coconut water

1 medium ripe papaya, peeled, seeded, and sliced

1 handful spinach

Instructions

Process all the ingredients in a juicer. Stir in coconut water. Serve and enjoy.

Calories 440; Protein 5.8 g; Sugar 73.3 g; Cholesterol 0 mg.

Apple and Pear Juice

Use this juice as a constipation remedy

Ingredients

1 apple

3 pears

Instructions

Process the apple and pears whole then serve.

Calories 313; Protein 1.8 g; Sugar 55.4 g; Cholesterol 0 mg.

Constipation Remedy Juice

Ingredients

3 tomatoes

2 cups of spinach

1 cup of broccoli heads

Instructions

First juice the broccoli and spinach as they produce less juice than the tomatoes. This will help flush the remaining broccoli and spinach juice out of the juicer into the glass or cup. Juice whole tomato for more nutrition. If you find it bitter, add lemon juice to taste.

Calories 262; Protein 23 g; Sugar .3 g; Cholesterol 0 mg.

Apple Kale Juice

Ingredients

2 granny smith apples

3 kale leaves with stalk

1 lime

1 lemon

1 red apple

1 inch ginger

Instructions

Juice all ingredients then serve.

Calories 307; Protein 6.2 g; Sugar 47.7 g; Cholesterol 0 mg.

Juicing Recipes for your Digestive System

Most think that the digestive system simply process food out of the body, but it really does much more than that. Within your digestive system, there are hormones released, enzymes created, toxins taken out, vitamins and minerals transported to their respective organs, and much more. If your digestive system is not working properly, you may have issues with sleep, bowel movement, allergies, and your metabolism. Add these juices to your line up to ensure your digestive system is running smoothly.

Fall Time Flush

Ingredients

2 organic red apples

2 organic plums

1 cup of organic raspberries

Instructions

Cut up the apples and plums into chunks if desired. Rinse the raspberries well. Process the raspberries, then plums and apples. Stir or shake and serve.

Calories 265; Protein 2.7 g; Sugar41.8 g; Cholesterol 0 mg.

Melon Mania

Ingredients

½ of honeydew melon

½ of cantaloupe

¼ of watermelon

Slice of lemon, to serve (optional)

Instructions

Cut up the melon, cantaloupe and watermelon into chunks. Process all of the ingredients, and service with a squeeze of lemon, if desired. Stir or shake and serve.

Calories 318; Protein 6.4 g; Sugar 69.4 g; Cholesterol 0 mg.

Kiwi Strawberry Juice

Ingredients

2 cups of organic strawberries

2 medium kiwis

2 organic green apples

Slice of lemon, to serve (optional)

Instructions

Peel the kiwis and rinse the strawberries thoroughly. Dice the apples if desired for ease of processing. Process the strawberries, then kiwi, and finally the apples. Service with a squeeze of lemon if desired. Stir or shake, then serve.

Calories 327; Protein 4.0 g; Sugar 44.7 g; Cholesterol 0 mg.

Papaya Pineapple Punch

Ingredients

½ of organic papaya

½ of pineapple

2 organic green apples

Slice of lemon, to serve (optional)

Instructions

Cube the pineapple, apples and papaya. Process the pineapple, followed by the papaya, and finally the apples. Add a squeeze of lemon to serve if desired. Stir or shake and serve.

Calories 405; Protein 3.6 g; Sugar 77.2 g; Cholesterol 0 mg.

Good Morning Mango

Ingredients

2 mangoes

2 organic green apples

2 pears

Instructions

Peel and cube the mangoes. Dice the apples and pears, as well. Process all of the fruits. Stir or shake and serve.

Calories 574; Protein 3.8 g; Sugar 117.3 g; Cholesterol 0 mg.

Peach and Pear Juice

Ingredients

2 plums

2 peaches

2 pears

Instructions

Dice all of the fruits and process together. Stir or shake and serve.

Calories 306; Protein 3.3 g; Sugar 58.6 g; Cholesterol 0 mg.

Cabbage Green Beet Juice

Ingredients

2 organic beets

2 medium carrots

1 cup of organic cabbage

1 cup of organic collard greens

Slice of lemon, to serve (optional)

Instructions

Cut up the beets and carrots into cubes, and lightly chop the collard greens and cabbage. Juice in this order for maximum juice: collard greens, beets, cabbage, carrots. Add a garnish of lemon or a squeeze of lemon to serve. Stir or shake and serve.

Calories 157; Protein 6.7 g; Sugar 16.8 g; Cholesterol 0 mg.

Juicing Recipes for Female Health

Hormones govern many processes of the body's systems, and their role in health cannot be denied. The below recipes are ideal for creating balance for the female hormones, and in turn her body's rhythms and systems.

Weight Loss Water

Ingredients

2 grapefruits, juiced in citrus juicer

1 lemon, juicer in citrus juicer

2 organic green apples

1 stalk of celery

Instructions

Juice the grapefruits and lemon in a citrus juicer and set aside. Process the apples and celery, and add the lemon and grapefruit juice. Stir or shake and serve.

Calories 309; Protein 3.0 g; Sugar 63.7 g; Cholesterol 0 mg.

Bloody Mary Juice

Ingredients

1 stalk of celery

3 medium tomatoes, or 3 cups of baby tomatoes

3 carrots

Slice of lemon to serve, optional

Instructions

Process the tomatoes, followed by the celery and carrots. Stir or shake and serve.

Calories 208; Protein 7.0 g; Sugar 9.8 g; Cholesterol 0 mg.

Hair and Nails Tonic

Ingredients

2 sweet potatoes

2 cups of butternut squash

3 carrots

Slice of lemon to serve, optional

Instructions

Dice the potatoes, squash and carrots. Process all ingredients. Garnish with lemon or a squeeze of lemon juice to serve if desired. Stir or shake and serve.

Calories 512; Protein 8.4 g; Sugar 9.7 g; Cholesterol 0 mg.

Mama's Everyday Juice

Ingredients

2 carrots

2 beets

2 prunes

2 organic green apples

Instructions

Dice all ingredients, then process in this order: prunes, beets, apples, carrots. Stir or shake and serve.

Calories 537; Protein 6.8 g; Sugar 108.6 g; Cholesterol 0 mg.

Coffee Replacement

Ingredients

1 cup of radish or broccoli sprouts

5 carrots

2 organic green apples

Slice of lime to serve, optional

Instructions

Dice the apples and carrots, then process the sprouts, followed by the apples and carrots. Stir or shake and serve.

Calories 278; Protein 5.0 g; Sugar 42.8 g; Cholesterol 0 mg.

Juicing Recipes for Male Health

Males have certain dietary and hormonal needs, and there are a number of fruits and vegetables which benefit the male health in particular. Juicing is the most effective and quickest way to deliver raw, whole food nutrition into your body to regulate its systems and produce health.

Prostate Boost Juice

Ingredients

3 medium tomatoes or 4 cups of baby tomatoes

2 stalks of celery

½ bunch of collard greens

2 carrots

Instructions

Dice the carrots for ease of processing. Process the tomatoes, followed by the collard greens, then celery and carrots. Stir or shake and serve.

Calories 218; Protein 7.6 g; Sugar 11.8 g; Cholesterol 0 mg.

Mean Green Male Juice

Ingredients

3 pieces of bok choy

1 stalk of celery

½ cup of organic kale

2 organic green apples

Instructions

Dice the apples. Process the kale, then bok choy, celery and apples. Stir and shake and serve.

Calories 197; Protein 5.9 g; Sugar 29.5 g; Cholesterol 0 mg.

Fiberful Morning Juice

Ingredients

½ head of cauliflower

½ head of cabbage

Juice of 1 lemon, juiced in citrus juicer

2 stalks of celery

2 carrots

Instructions

Chop the carrots for ease of processing. Process the cabbage, followed by the cauliflower, then the celery and carrot. Add the lemon juice. Stir or shake and serve.

Calories 173; Protein 8.8 g; Sugar 6.3 g; Cholesterol 0 mg.

Berry Blast for Men

Ingredients

2 cups of organic strawberries

1 cups of organic raspberries

1 cups of organic blueberries

½ bunch of organic kale

Instructions

Chop the apples and carrots for ease of processing. Process all the berries, followed by the kale. Stir or shake and serve.

Calories 185; Protein 4.7 g; Sugar 17.9 g; Cholesterol 0 mg.

Juicing Recipes For Kids

It's difficult to get all of the nutrients children need daily in their diet. Though you can supplement, most commercially-made vitamins and minerals are synthetic, and may do more harm than good. Juices are an excellent way to deliver large quantities of vitamins and minerals to your little one, without them even knowing. Juices are also vibrant and colorful, making children excited to give them a try.

Unfortunately, the majority of the food marketed to children today is full of toxic preservatives, pesticides, and food dyes. All of these processed items slow down the child's digestion, cause eczema, allergies and asthma, and even behavioral or autoimmune conditions. If your child is suffering from bowel or stomach issues, behavioral problems, or any autoimmune issue, such as eczema, then clearing the diet of all glutinous grains and sugars, as well as removing preservatives, pesticides, and food dyes, is advised. Adding juices can quickly turn around the body's ability to heal these issues, and help detox from the effects of processed toxins.

Involving kids in the process of juicing will make the small task of drinking them even more exciting, as well as educational. Kids can learn the names of fruits and vegetables, practice their colors, learn how plants grow, and maybe even help clean up.

Purple Juice

Ingredients

2 beets

1 prune

2 organic green apples

Instructions

Process the prune, followed by the beets and apples. Stir or shake and serve.

Calories 396; Protein 4.9 g; Sugar 81.9 g; Cholesterol 0 mg.

Green Juice

Ingredients

3 stalks of celery

2 organic green apples

2 cups of organic spinach

Instructions

Juice the spinach, followed by the celery and apples. Stir or shake and serve.

Calories 188; Protein 3.8 g; Sugar 29 g; Cholesterol 0 mg.

Citrus Morning Juice

Ingredients

1 orange, juiced in citrus juicer

1 lemon or lime, juiced in citrus juicer

3 carrots

1 cup of filtered water

Instructions

Juice the orange and lemon or lime in citrus juicer, set aside. Juice the carrots, and add the citrus juice with one cup of filtered water. Stir or shake and serve.

Calories 152; Protein 3.2 g; Sugar 22.3g; Cholesterol 0 mg.

Gentle Detox Juice

Ingredients

1 cup of fresh, organic parsley

1 cup of fresh, organic cilantro

4 carrots

Instructions

Juice the parsley and cilantro, followed by the carrots.

Calories 122; Protein 4.5 g; Sugar 11.9 g; Cholesterol 0 mg.

Orange Julius Juice

Ingredients

5 carrots

1 orange, juiced in citrus juicer

2 peaches

Instructions

Juice the orange in the citrus juicer and set aside. Juice the peaches, followed by the carrots.

Calories 271; Protein 5.6g; Sugar 44.5 g; Cholesterol 0 mg.

Juicing Recipes For Brain Fog

Many people report low energy and brain fog. Recent studies show that a diet rich in fruits and vegetables, healthy fats like Omega 3's, and whole grains, helps prevent diseases such as Alzheimer's. Ensuring that your diet is rich in vitamins and minerals can help keep brain fog and brain diseases at bay. Often, minor issues are the result of mineral deficiencies. Sugars and simple starches can also cause havoc on the brain if consumed in high quantities. If you have periods where you struggle to concentrate, try to limit your simple carbohydrate consumption, such as white bread and rice, sugars, and candies. Try these recipes first thing in the morning to beat off the brain fog without coffee.

Morning Coffee

Ingredients

1 teaspoon ground cayenne pepper

4 cloves of garlic

½ cup of apple cider vinegar

1 cup of filtered water

Instructions

Warm the filtered water, and chop or grind the garlic. Add the apple cider vinegar, cayenne pepper, and garlic to the water. Stir and enjoy.

Calories 24; Protein 1 g; Sugar.3 g; Cholesterol 0 mg.

Good Fat Drink

Ingredients

1 tablespoon of coconut oil

1 avocado

1 cup of spinach

2 organic green apples

Instructions

Blend the coconut oil and avocado in a blender or in a bowl with fork. Juice the spinach and green apples. Combine the two mixtures, and shake well.

Calories 709; Protein 8.7 g; Sugar 51.6 g; Cholesterol 0 mg.

Brain Power Punch

Ingredients

2 cups of kale

2 cups of spinach

2 cups of blueberries

Instructions

Juice the kale and spinach, followed by the berries. Stir or shake and serve.

Calories 249; Protein 8.7 g; Sugar 33.5 g; Cholesterol 0 mg.

Purple Brain Power

Ingredients

3 beets

2 prunes

2 carrots

Instructions

Process the prunes, followed by the beets and carrots. Stir or shake and serve.

Calories 338; Protein 6.7 g; Sugar 64.3 g; Cholesterol 0 mg.

Nighttime Brain Calmer

Ingredients

2 cups of dark cherries, pitted

2 carrots

2 stalks of celery

Instructions

Pit the cherries, and process, followed by the carrots and celery. Stir and enjoy!

Calories 218; Protein 4.6 g; Sugar 35.6 g; Cholesterol 0 mg.

Juice Recipes For Specific Illnesses And Diseases

Chronic illness is skyrocketing in modern societies. Recent reports show that up to half of children in developed countries have at least one type of chronic illness, and those numbers keep climbing. Some children are even on multiple prescriptions, and the majority of people by middle age will be on at least one prescription. While genetics can play a role, epigenetics tells us that what we put in our bodies greatly affects how our bodies perform. What you put in, truly does come out. People suffering with nearly every disease report less pain and better function after incorporating more plant-based foods into their diet, and juicing is the most effective way to do so.

Juice Recipe for Diabetes

Ingredients

2 organic green apples

2 carrots

2 cups of broccoli

Instructions

Juice the broccoli, followed by the apples and carrots. Stir or shake and serve.

Calories 243; Protein 7.1 g; Sugar 34.3 g; Cholesterol 0 mg.

Juice Recipe for Heart Disease

Ingredients

2 cups of broccoli

2 organic green apples

2 cups of blueberries or mulberries

Instructions

Process the berries, followed by the broccoli, and finally the apples. Stir or shake and serve.

Calories 355; Protein 7.9 g; Sugar 58.7 g; Cholesterol 0 mg.

Juice Recipe for Inflammation

Ingredients

1 ginger root

1 turmeric root

2 cups of spinach

1 cup of filtered water, if desired

½ cup of apple cider vinegar, if desired

Instructions

Juice the ginger and turmeric root, followed by the spinach. Drink as is, or add filtered water and apple cider vinegar for further benefits, if desired. Stir and enjoy.

Calories 61; Protein 2.8 g; Sugar .8 g; Cholesterol 0 mg.

Juice Recipe for Arthritis

Ingredients

2 carrots

2 cups of broccoli

1 cup of cherries

Instructions

Juice the cherries, followed by the broccoli and carrots. Stir or shake and serve.

Calories 173; Protein 7.7 g; Sugar 20.6g; Cholesterol 0 mg.

Juice Recipe for Joint Issues

Ingredients

2 sweet potatoes

2 carrots

Instructions

Juice the potatoes, followed by the carrots. Stir or shake and serve.

Calories 153; Protein 3.6 g; Sugar 14.5 g; Cholesterol 0 mg.

Juice Recipe for Sleep Issues

Ingredients

2 cups of dark red cherries

1 cup of grapes

1 cup of filtered water, if desired

Instructions

Juice the cherries, followed by the grapes. Drink as is, or add a cup of filtered water for taste. Stir and enjoy before bed.

Calories 322; Protein 5.2 g; Sugar 5.6 g; Cholesterol 0 mg.

Juice Recipe for Digestive Issues

Ingredients

2 organic green apples

3 carrots

2 cups of cilantro

Instructions

Process the cilantro, followed by the apples and carrots. Stir or shake and serve.

Calories 219; Protein 2.8 g; Sugar 37.3 g; Cholesterol 0 mg.

Juice Recipe for Constipation

Ingredients

4 prunes

1 cup of filtered water

1/8 teaspoon of pink Himalayan sea salt

1 tablespoon of coconut oil, optional

Instructions

Juice the prunes, and add the sea salt and water. Add a tablespoon of coconut oil, if desired. You may need to warm the coconut oil so it will mix well. Stir and enjoy.

Calories 119; Protein .7 g; Sugar 12.8 g; Cholesterol 0 mg.

Juice Recipe for Heart Burn

Ingredients

2 ginger roots

2 cups of kale

1 cup of filtered water

Instructions

Juice the ginger and kale, and add the water if desired. For a warm drink, warm the water before pouring into the juice. Stir and enjoy.

Calories 82; Protein 5.1 g; Sugar 3.4 g; Cholesterol 0 mg.

Juice Recipe for Headaches

Ingredients

2 cups of Swiss chard

2 cups of spinach

1 banana

Instructions

Juice the chard and spinach, and mash the banana in a bowl. Combine the two ingredients, adding a bit of filtered water if desired. Stir and enjoy.

Calories 249; Protein 10.7 g; Sugar 31.7 g; Cholesterol 0 mg.

10 Day Cleanse

Your body is a machine that needs to rest and reboot at times. Cleansing the body seasonally, that is at the changes of the seasons, has been an age-old recipe for longevity and radiant health. If you are suffering from a chronic condition or inflammation, poor digestion, low energy, or any other ailment, it is a good idea to complete a cleanse before you begin any diet or lifestyle changes, so that you get off to the right start. A cleanse helps your body release toxins, which in turns allows your digestive and other organs to function properly. After a cleanse, your metabolism will be functioning better, and your digestion will improve to grab even more of the vitamins and minerals you consume (maybe from juice!) and shuttle them to your organs. When cleansing the body, it's best to work from the bottom to the top. You do not want to first detox the small intestine with a congested, toxin-laden colon. Toxins would build up in your colon and possibly not be able to pass, creating more havoc than at first. Therefore, begin with Day One and following the cleanse Days exactly.

Cleanse Tips

- Drink this cleanse in order to ensure you are detoxing properly.
- Incorporate the below juices into your daily regimen, and eat two other meals that day. Most find it best to have a juice for breakfast, with the other two as snacks before or after lunch and dinner.
- Try to eat meals with limited meats, butters, and oils, as these will slow the detoxification process.
- Drink at least 8 cups of filtered water daily during the cleanse. Sipping on warm water instead of cold will also improve digestion and cleansing.
- Try to avoid all cold beverages and treats, including slushies, shakes, and ice creams.
- Try to limit soy, dairy, and refined starches (white bread, white rice, crackers) during the cleanse.

Day 1 Cleanse – Juicing Recipes for Colon Detoxification

Juicing Recipe 1

Ingredients

3 organic green apples

7 carrots

Instructions

Chop up the apples and carrots for easier processing, and juice both. Stir or shake and serve.

Calories 390; Protein 5.2 g; Sugar 62.7 g; Cholesterol 0 mg.

Juicing Recipe 2

Ingredients

1 organic green apple

2 carrots

½ head of cauliflower

½ head of broccoli

Instructions

Chop the apple and carrots for easier processing. Break apart the broccoli and cauliflower and process. Then, process the apple and carrots. Stir or shake and serve.

Calories 221; Protein 2.1 g; Sugar 20.0 g; Cholesterol 0 mg.

Juicing Recipe 3

Ingredients

2 sweet potatoes

1 cup of chopped pumpkin

2 organic green apples

2 carrots

Instructions

Chop all of the ingredients into cubes. Process the pumpkin, sweet potatoes, apples and then carrots. Stir or shake and serve.

Calories 516; Protein 5.9 g; Sugar 36.8 g; Cholesterol 0 mg.

Day 2 Cleanse – Juicing Recipes for Large Intestine Detoxification

Juicing Recipe 1

Ingredients

2 pears

2 organic green apples

4 carrots

Slice of lemon to serve, optional

Instructions

Dice up the pears, apples and carrots for ease of processing. Juice the pears, followed by the apples and carrots. Garnish with lemon, or squeeze a bit of lemon into the juice. Stir or shake, and serve.

Calories 380; Protein 3.5 g; Sugar 64.5 g; Cholesterol 0 mg.

Juicing Recipe 2

Ingredients

1 cup of spinach

3 carrots

2 organic green apples

2 tablespoons of psyllium husks

Instructions

Juice the spinach, followed by the carrots and green apples. Add the psyllium husks and stir. Drink immediately, as the psyllium husks will make the drink spongey over time. Stir and serve.

Calories 275; Protein 3.3 g; Sugar 37.5 g; Cholesterol 0 mg.

Juicing Recipe 3

Ingredients

3 carrots

2 organic green apples

½ head of broccoli

2 pears

Instructions

Dice up the pears, apples and carrots for ease in processing. Break off pieces of the broccoli, and process. Then, process the pears, followed by the apples and carrots. Stir or shake, and serve.

Calories 465; Protein 12.5 g; Sugar 64.5 g; Cholesterol 0 mg.

Day 3 Cleanse – Juicing Recipes for Small Intestine Detoxification

Juicing Recipe 1

Ingredients

2 prunes

4 stalks of asparagus

2 organic green apples

3 carrots

Instructions

Cut up the apples, carrots, asparagus and prunes into chunks for ease of processing. Process the prunes, followed by the asparagus, and finally the apples and carrots. Stir or shake and serve.

Calories 506; Protein 6.3 g; Sugar 100.3 g; Cholesterol 0 mg.

Juicing Recipe 2

Ingredients

2 organic green apples

2 sweet potatoes

10 carrots

Instructions

Cut up the apples, potatoes and carrots into chunks for ease of processing. Process the potatoes, followed by the apples and carrots. Stir or shake and serve.

Calories 254 ; Protein 5 g; Sugar 24 g; Cholesterol 0 mg.

Juicing Recipe 3

Ingredients

10-12 brussel sprouts

2 organic green apples

3 carrots

2 pears

Slice of lemon to serve, optional

Instructions

Cut up the apples, carrots and pears for ease of processing. Process the pears, followed by the brussel sprouts. Then, juice the apples and carrots. Garnish with lemon to serve, or a squeeze of lemon juice. Stir or shake and serve.

Calories 425; Protein 6.5 g; Sugar 66.5 g; Cholesterol 0 mg.

Day 4 Cleanse – Juicing Recipes for Overall Detoxification

As your body is flushing out and possibly detoxing from sugars, starch, and other unhealthy foods, this cleanse day will be simple.

Juicing Recipe 1

Ingredients

2 organic green apples

3 carrots

½ bunch of spinach

Slice of lemon to serve, optional

Instructions

Dice the apples and carrots for ease of processing. Process the spinach, followed by the apples and carrots. Garnish with a slice of lemon, or squeeze of lemon juice. Stir or shake, and serve.

Calories 235; Protein 3.3 g; Sugar 37.5 g; Cholesterol 0 mg.

Juicing Recipe 2

Ingredients

3 beets

3 carrots

2 organic green apples

Instructions

Dice the beets, carrots and apples, and process all ingredients. Stir or shake and serve.

Calories 324; Protein 6.4 g; Sugar 53.7 g; Cholesterol 0 mg.

Juicing Recipe 3

Ingredients

½ bunch of kale

½ bunch of spinach

2 organic green apples

3 carrots

Instructions

Dice the apples and carrots. Process the greens, followed by the apples and carrots. Stir or shake and serve.

Calories 262; Protein 5.8g; Sugar 38.9 g; Cholesterol 0 mg.

Day 5 Cleanse – Juicing Recipes for Pancreas Detoxification

Juicing Recipe 1

Ingredients

2 cups of organic blueberries

½ bunch of spinach

2 organic green apples

3 carrots

Instructions

Dice the apples and carrots. Process the blueberries, followed by the spinach, and then the apples and carrots. Stir or shake and serve.

Calories 266; Protein 3.6 g; Sugar 44.7 g; Cholesterol 0 mg.

Juicing Recipe 2

Ingredients

2 cups of red grapes

2 organic green apples

3 carrots

2 cups of pineapple

Instructions

Dice the apples and carrots. Process the grapes, followed by the pineapple, then the apples and carrots. Stir or shake and serve.

Calories 495; Protein 9.7 g; Sugar 99.1 g; Cholesterol 0 mg.

Juicing Recipe 3

Ingredients

2 medium tomatoes, or 3 cups of baby tomatoes

3 carrots

½ head of broccoli

Instructions

Dice up the carrots for ease of processing. Process the tomatoes, followed by the broccoli, then carrots. Stir or shake and serve.

Calories 237; Protein 8.4 g; Sugar 14.0 g; Cholesterol 0 mg.

Day 6 Cleanse – Juicing Recipes for Gallbladder Detoxification

Juicing Recipe 1

Ingredients

½ head of cauliflower

2 organic green apples

1 stalk of celery

Instructions

Dice the apples for ease of processing. Process the cauliflower, followed by the celery and apples. Stir or shake and serve.

Calories 226; Protein 6.8 g; Sugar 28.7g; Cholesterol 0 mg.

Juicing Recipe 2

Ingredients

3 cups of pineapple

1 cup of papaya

1 cup of organic spinach

Instructions

Dice the papaya for ease of processing. Process the papaya, followed by the spinach, and finally the pineapple. Stir or shake and serve.

Calories 290; Protein 3.5 g; Sugar 56.4 g; Cholesterol 0 mg.

Juicing Recipe 3

Ingredients

3 carrots

2 organic green apples

1 cup of papaya

2 cups of cherries (of choice)

Instructions

Dice the papaya, carrots and apples for ease of processing. Process the cherries, followed by the papaya, then apples and carrots. Stir or shake and serve.

Calories 391; Protein 3.1 g; Sugar 69.5 g; Cholesterol 0 mg.

Day 7 Cleanse – Juicing Recipes for Liver Detoxification

Juicing Recipe 1

Ingredients

1 grapefruit, juiced in citrus juicer

2 organic green apples

3 carrots

Instructions

Juice one grapefruit in a citrus juicer, set aside. Juice the apples and carrots, then add the juice of the grapefruit. Stir or shake and serve.

Calories 263; Protein 3.7 g; Sugar 48.4 g; Cholesterol 0 mg.

Juicing Recipe 2

Ingredients

1 cup of cabbage

1 cup of cauliflower

2 beets

3 carrots

Slice of lemon to serve, optional

Instructions

Chop the cauliflower or cabbage, and dice the beets and carrots. Process the cabbage, followed by the cauliflower, and finally the carrots. Stir or shake and serve.

Calories 193; Protein 7.7 g; Sugar 19.5 g; Cholesterol 0 mg.

Juicing Recipe 3

Ingredients

2 limes, squeezed or juiced in citrus juicer

1 cup of broccoli

1 cup of spinach

2 organic green apples

Instructions

Juice the lime in a citrus juicer and set aside. Process the broccoli, followed by the spinach, and finally the apples. Add the lime juice, and stir or shake and serve.

Calories 149; Protein 2.6 g; Sugar 29.3 g; Cholesterol 0 mg.

Day 8 Cleanse – Juicing Recipes for Blood Detoxification

Juicing Recipe 1

Ingredients

2 apricots

2 prunes

1 cup of watermelon

2 organic green apples

1 cup of mulberries, if available

Instructions

Core and chop the apricots, and chop up the prunes, and apples for ease of processing. Process the watermelon, followed by the prunes, mulberries, and apricots, and finally the apples.

Calories 298; Protein 4.9 g; Sugar 57.2 g; Cholesterol 0 mg.

Juicing Recipe 2

Ingredients

2 beets

3 carrots

2 organic green apples

Instructions

Dice the beets, carrots and apples for ease of processing. Process the beets, carrots, then apples. Stir or shake and serve.

Calories 260; Protein 5.0 g; Sugar 42.4 g; Cholesterol 0 mg.

Juicing Recipe 3

Ingredients

2 beets

1 cup organic spinach

1 cup organic kale

2 carrots

Instructions

Dice the beets and carrots for ease of processing. Process the kale and spinach, and then the beets and carrots. Stir or shake and serve.

Calories 189; Protein 7.8 g; Sugar 21.2 g; Cholesterol 0 mg.

Day 9 Cleanse – Juicing Recipes for Endocrine Detoxification

Juicing Recipe 1

Ingredients

2 sweet potatoes

2 turnips

3 carrots

1 cup of organic kale

Instructions

Dice the potatoes, turnips and carrots for ease of processing. Process the kale, then turnips, sweet potatoes and carrots. Stir or shake and serve.

Calories 453; Protein 10.8 g; Sugar 19.3 g; Cholesterol 0mg.

Juicing Recipe 2

Ingredients

1 bunch (about 12 pieces) of asparagus

2 organic green apples

1 cup of mustard greens (or collard greens)

3 carrots

Slice of lemon to serve, optional

Instructions

Dice the apples and carrots for ease of processing. Process the greens, followed by the asparagus, and finally the apples and carrots. Garnish with a lemon slice, or squeeze of lemon juice. Stir or shake and serve.

Calories 284; Protein 10.0 g; Sugar 37.2 g; Cholesterol 0 mg.

Juicing Recipe 3

Ingredients

1 cup of mulberries, if available

1 cup of organic raspberries

1 cup of organic strawberries

1 cup of organic spinach

3 carrots

Instructions

Dice the carrots for ease of processing. Process the berries, then the spinach, and finally the apple and carrots. Stir or shake and serve.

Calories 248; Protein 6.7 g; Sugar 27.9 g; Cholesterol 0 mg.

Day 10 Cleanse – Juicing Recipes for Overall Detoxification

Juicing Recipe 1

Ingredients

2 beets

3 carrots

2 organic green apples

Slice of lemon to serve, optional

Instructions

Dice the beets, carrots and apples. Process all ingredients, and serve with a garnish of lemon or squeeze of lemon juice if desired. Stir or shake and serve.

Calories 289; Protein 5.1 g; Sugar 28.2 g; Cholesterol 0 mg.

Juicing Recipe 2

Ingredients

1 cup of organic kale

1 cup of organic spinach

1 cup of collard greens

1 sweet potato

3 carrots

Instructions

Dice the potato and carrots for ease of processing. Process the kale, spinach, and greens, followed by the potato and carrots. Stir or shake and serve.

Calories 285; Protein 9.3 g; Sugar 10.2 g; Cholesterol 0mg.

Juicing Recipe 3

Ingredients

2 pears

2 cups of pineapple

2 organic green apples

1 stalk of celery

Instructions

Dice the apples and pears for ease of processing. Process the pears, pineapple, then apples and celery. Stir or shake and serve.

Calories 484; Protein 4.1 g; Sugar 91.6 g; Cholesterol 0 mg.

After your Cleanse

Great job! You more than likely lost some weight, gained some energy, and feel wonderful after finishing your cleanse. Now you can slowly add back in more meats, oils, nuts, and dairy. Do not lose the benefits of your cleanse by adding back too many unhealthy foods. Maintain your cleanse benefits by eating healthy as often as possible, and keeping a juice in your diet 4-5 days per week.

Conclusion

I am sure with all the amazing green juicing recipes outlined in this book, you are ready to start taking green juices for a healthier you. Not all juice combinations will fit your taste buds. However, don't worry since you can try out different juices and combinations of vegetables and fruits until you can find what works for you.

Juicing is one of the most effective and efficient ways to deliver key nutrients to your body's cells and organs. Those who juice regularly report that they have increased stamina, energy, and are generally healthier. Here's to a healthier you!

www.ingramcontent.com/pod-product-compliance
Lightning Source LLC
Chambersburg PA
CBHW072103280526
45788CB00006B/2381